AF417302

HEALTHY CHILDREN: FOOD, EXERCISE, STRESS MANAGEMENT AND USE OF TECHNOLOGY

HEALTHY CHILDREN

FOOD, EXERCISE, STRESS MANAGEMENT AND USE OF TECHNOLOGY

INDEX

Introduction

The need to ensure the health of children is one of the most important obligations of parents. In today's world, where many adults tend to live an unhealthy and inactive lifestyle, it is crucial to teach children the essentials of health while they are young. Get all the information you need in this book!

Let's get started!

Chapter 1: Introduction

While you can still guide them, you have to help them understand the different aspects of their health.

In doing this, you don't have to sound like you're giving a sermon or a lecture.

By raising and caring for them along with their other daily activities, you can ensure that your children have a healthy and balanced lifestyle.

Basically

Developing the right habits

The habits that children would develop will surely be maintained throughout their adulthood. While they are young, it is every parent's duty to help them develop the right habits. Along with character development, children's daily habits should also be taken into account, for example, the foods they eat, their physical activities, their relationships with other people, and even their perceptions about things and the environment.

Children do not have a broad knowledge of the world. Most of the time, they are easily tempted by food or even by activities that they find fun and enjoyable without considering the negative effects.

To help them, it is necessary to discipline your children in such a way that they grow up to become responsible, health-conscious and mature individuals.

Healthy Diet

Many, if not all, parents will have trouble feeding their children. After all, even adults have difficulty eating a healthy diet for the main reason that in doing so, they have to eat nutritious but bland foods.

Children's appetites can be very sensitive. Young children are often easily attracted to eating foods that contain too much oil, such as fried chicken, potato chips, etc. Several children cannot refuse to eat chocolates, candies and other products that contain too much sugar. There is really nothing wrong with this. But anything that is too much can also be dangerous. As a parent, you must control the foods your children eat. There are ways to provide them with creative foods that are both delicious and nutritious.

Physical Activity

In addition to their daily eating habits, children also need to exercise. Considering their age, you can't force them to exercise if they don't want to. For sports or other activities that involve playing with other kids, you can make sure your children are physically active. Not only do you enjoy the company of other children, but your child also has the opportunity to exercise without his or her knowledge.

Learn these tips

This is basically the main purpose of this book, to provide a holistic approach and insightful advice to ensure the good health of your children. The book is divided into different chapters covering balanced diet, exercise and even stress. With these helpful tips, recipes, and other important information, you will have the opportunity to learn more about the different dimensions of your children's health.

Chapter 2: What Young People Need for a Healthy Diet

To ensure that your children have a complete and well-balanced diet, you need to know the specific types of foods they need to eat along with the right amount of vitamins and minerals they need.

Many parents have general knowledge about what foods they should eat and what foods they should avoid.

But you also need to know the right portion to target the full amount of vitamins and minerals the body needs.

What do they need?

Dietary Guidelines for Young Children

Young children need to have the full amount of nutrition for their growth and development. As a parent, it is helpful to know the dietary guidelines so you can prepare the right foods for them.

Whole grain cereals: In the morning, you can eat bread or buckwheat pancakes. In the evening, you can include brown rice for dinner. Just make sure your children get four servings of whole grains a day.

Fruits and vegetables: Your children should eat two servings of fruits and vegetables every day. In the morning, they can eat apples or other snacks containing fruit. You can also make soups using nutritious vegetables.

Protein: Children need protein to build their muscles. In one day, you need to have two servings. Encourage your children to eat eggs, fish, lamb, chicken and baked beans.

Milk and dairy products: For your child's bone development, you need to provide three servings. Your child can eat cheese, milk, yogurt, etc.

Vitamins and minerals: Using supplements can also help ensure that your child gets the right amount of vitamins and minerals.

Nutritional Guidelines for School-Aged Children

As children grow, they will need to eat more and have the nutrition that adults need. From eating whole grains (oats, rice, millet, etc.) to healthy fruits, vegetables, and protein, your children also need to have healthy fats, including the following:

Monounsaturated fats: Avocados, canola oil, peanut oil, sesame seeds, etc.

Trans fats: This type is found in cookies,

crackers, margarines, etc.

Polyunsaturated fats: Omega-3 fatty acids (good for the heart) and Omega-6 fatty acids such as salmon, sardines, anchovies, nuts and more.

Dietary guidelines

Whole grains: School-aged children should take 6 to 11 servings of whole grains every day.

Fruits: For fruits, you should provide 2-4 servings in a day that may include ¾ cup of any fruit juice or ½ cup of sliced fruit.

Vegetables: 3- 5 servings are needed in a day. You may serve 3/5 cup of vegetable juice or 1 cup of leaf vegetables.

Dairy Products: 2-3 servings of yogurt, milk or natural cheese.

Zinc: To increase school performance and improve memory capacity, it is essential to have zinc which is found in beef, pork, liver, milk, cocoa and poultry among many others.

Prepare sumptuous and nutritious meals

Encouraging your child to eat nutritious meals is a difficult task, especially if your child has sensitive food preferences. To ensure that the vitamins and minerals are complete, be creative with the foods you prepare and always keep in mind that you should prepare delicious meals.

Chapter 3: What foods to keep away from children

Children love sweets and other foods that lack nutritional value. Since the foods your children eat can definitely impact their growth and development, it is essential to know which specific foods to avoid. Knowing what kinds of food products and foods to avoid can help guide your children when it comes to the food they eat.

Of course, you can't control your children's activities 24/7, especially if they're in school. But while they're young, you should help them develop the right eating habits.

Keep them away from these...

Limit sugar

All users had our childhood experiences of eating different candies and chocolates. For the children, they are happiest when they get to have these delicious sweets and chocolates. There is nothing wrong with letting your children eat candy. But you should make sure they don't overdo it. According to the American Heart Association, children are limited to 12 grams per day or 3 teaspoons per day.

There are ways to reduce sugar intake. For one thing, you can use less sugar when preparing and cooking meals. Another option is to avoid drinking sugary beverages such as soda and soft drinks. Instead, you can replace nutritious shakes. Finally, you should not allow your children to eat processed foods.

Reduce consumption of products with salt

Sodium is also necessary for the body. But children cannot consume too much salt. One teaspoon of salt already equals 2,300 mg of sodium.

There are guidelines for the maximum recommended salt intake for young children. For children ages 1-3, the maximum salt intake is 1,500 mg per day. Children 4-8 years of age should consume no more than 1,900 mg of sodium per day. For children 9-13 years old, the maximum salt intake is set at 2,200 mg per day.

How do you limit your salt intake?

There are several ways to reduce salt intake. Today, many children love going to restaurants and fast food. Most of these establishments use too much sodium.

To reduce your salt intake, it is strongly recommended that you prepare your meals at home rather than going to fast food restaurants.

It is also recommended to eat fresh vegetables instead of canned vegetables.

When you buy produce, you should choose low-salt products.

Avoid eating junk food

Junk food is everywhere. I'm sure your kids would like to eat different kinds of junk food, too.

These products have no nutritional value and some of them even contain too much salt and sugar. Therefore, you should encourage your children to avoid eating junk food, or if that's not possible, at least they can cut down on their junk food intake.

There are different alternatives that are more nutritious. For example, instead of eating chips, your children can eat graham crackers, fruit sauces, bagels, and English muffins.

Instead of eating ice cream, your kids can enjoy low-fat frozen yogurt or even fruit smoothies.

Chapter 4: Easy Ways to Get Kids to Eat Right

Children should have a healthy diet because they need certain vitamins and minerals to help them grow. With the right kind of diet, they can further develop their bodies, sharpen their minds, and become more energetic and physically active.

Unfortunately, this is easier said than done since many parents have to deal with different problems in this regard. On the one hand, young people still need to be guided as to which foods are healthy and which are not. Second, most children's natural tendency is to love foods that contain too much sugar, such as chocolates and candy. Third, it is part of their youth that they enjoy unhealthy foods such as junk food and other oily foods.

Do it the easy way

Developing the right eating habits

It is important that you help them develop the right eating habits.

You can still allow your children to eat chocolates, fried chicken, etc. But you must make sure they eat more nutritious meals and get the full vitamins and minerals their bodies need.

How exactly do their eating habits develop?

Eating regularly at home: Children need to know when it is the right time to eat and what foods they should eat. When you cook meals at home, you know that the ingredients used are healthy, unlike if you allow your children to eat fast food or buy food in the dining room. Prepare meals at home so you can easily control the food they eat.

Allow them to participate: Children want to participate too. When you go to the grocery store, you can take your children with you and let them select the items they can have for their lunchbox. Just monitor and sort the items they will choose and help them understand why they should avoid unhealthy food products.

Prepare healthy but nutritious meals: One of the main reasons kids hate to eat nutritious foods is that some prepare meals that are not visually appealing and lack taste. To entice your kids to eat healthy foods, you can search for certain recipes online that allow you to prepare foods with nutritional content without compromising taste. Be creative when preparing any meal. For example, you may want to use some art techniques just to make a meal visually appealing.

Encourage them to eat more fruits and vegetables. Every morning, you can make fresh, enjoyable smoothies that your kids are sure to love. Vegetables can also be used in different meals without them knowing it.

Avoid serving meals in large portions. The number of children who are obese is increasing over the years. This can be a serious problem if neglected. To avoid having to experience this type of problem, you should serve the right portion of each meal.

If you notice that your children tend to eat more than a normal child would, then you should seriously consider curbing their appetite to prevent them from gaining weight.

Chapter 5: What young people need for exercise

Just like adults, children need to exercise too. Aside from the importance of socializing and interacting with others, children develop their physical health when they exercise regularly.

Encouraging your children to exercise is not that difficult, since most children enjoy playing and being active. They like to run and have fun with other kids. These physical activities can now be considered exercise.

Your children can try different exercises and

activities. Depending on their own preferences, they can choose any activity they want.

Exercise

Importance of motivation

Most children are active and the natural tendency is to want to be playful most of the time. However, there are also children whose personalities are quite different. Some prefer to stay home and do activities that do not involve too much physical movement.

When this happens, the first thing young people need to exercise is motivation. This is also one of the most difficult things to do, especially if the children are not interested at all.

But with patience, parents can find ways to motivate their children to exercise.

Allocate time for exercise

When children are busy at school and have different activities they need to do, it is important for parents to take care of their daily schedules and make sure there is time for exercise.

By assigning one hour in a day, your children can already exercise.

Sports and other physical activities

Playing sports is one of the most effective types of exercise programs for your children. Not only do they develop self-discipline, but they also develop a person's overall health. You can enroll your child in a taekwondo class or other sports that interest him or her. Before he attends the class, you should buy the necessary items for him, including his taekwondo uniform, for example.

For girls, you can enroll your child in a skating class or ballet school. Children who sign up for a skating class need to have the proper equipment as well as the ice skates.

Children who are in the dance class need

dance shoes. Having the right attire allows them to perform better and enjoy their classes.

The most important thing to consider when choosing any activity is your child's interest. What are the things they like to do?

Tools and equipment

There are physical activities that may require certain tools and equipment. For example, there are children who want to try other sports such as cycling, ice hockey, and other activities that would require certain tools and equipment.

Parents with children who are enthusiastic

about these activities should definitely support them. Later, these hobbies may develop and children may begin to develop their passion.

Parents really need to invest in their children. Although they may have to part with some money just to ensure that they work on their physical health, at least they will be able to provide for their children's needs.

Of course, there are also other ways that kids can exercise without having to spend so much.

Chapter 6: Easy Ways to Get Kids to Exercise

Young people also need to exercise regularly to help them develop the different aspects of their health. Considering that vitality comes at an early age, children are naturally active and playful. Therefore, they will not encounter any difficulties in this regard. When they run and play with other children, they already have the opportunity to exercise.

But on the other hand, there are also children who are not so active. There are other children who are quite shy and who are not really into physical activities. Some children prefer to try other activities where they can't exercise.

If this is the case, parents should find ways to get their children to exercise. This can be a challenge if your child doesn't want to do too much physical activity.

Get them moving

How do you do it?

1. Allow children to socialize.

For children to exercise, you don't have to force them or make them do the usual adult exercise programs. There are many children who like to play in kindergartens and playgrounds. Even if your child is not physically active, he or she can interact with other children. Playing with friends is already a form of exercise. There is nothing better than the fun of running and playing with other children.

2. Encourage children to try sports.

Any sporting activity is not just for adults. Even children can try different types of sports depending on their preferences. From swimming, tae kwon do, table tennis to skating, they can choose the sport they want to try.

There are several benefits to be gained when

children practice an active sport. On the one hand, it is the best form of exercise, especially when children try very physical sports such as swimming, judo, taekwondo and athletics, among many others. Secondly, sports also help children develop a sense of responsibility. They begin to mature and are more disciplined. Sports help form and develop a child's personality and character. This is one of the reasons why so many parents want to enroll their children in different sports activities.

3. Parents should join their children in making physical activities more fun.

From time to time, parents can join their children in any physical activity they do. When children see their mom or dad playing with them, they feel more motivated. Parents also have the opportunity to bond and spend quality time with their children. Each weekend, you can plan different activities for your kids and let them have fun. There are many things you can share with your children where they have the opportunity to exercise their bodies.

4. Try the indoor activities.

For kids who really don't want to go out much, there are indoor activities they can try. There are game consoles where kids can move around and get some exercise. Parents can also invest in different tools and equipment where children can exercise even if they are at home.

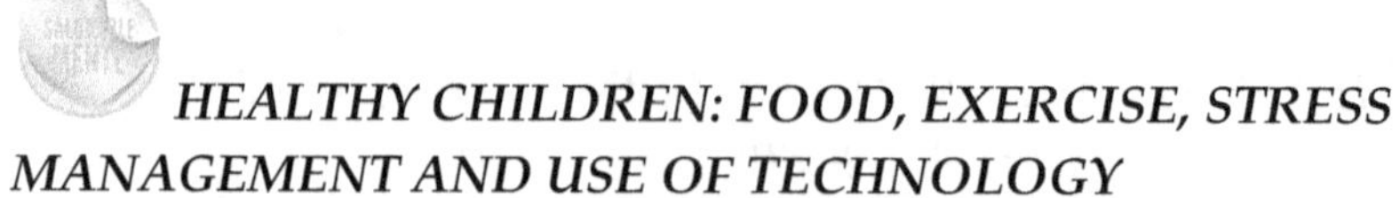

Chapter 7: The Impact of Stress on Children

Stress is one of the main factors that cause many people to contract certain diseases and illnesses. Although adults are more likely to experience stress from work, lifestyle, and personal relationships, children are not immune either. There are many factors that can contribute to stress. At home or even at school, children can experience stress.

With the intricate relationships people have today and the type of environment that surrounds them, it's difficult to protect your children from stressful situations. That's why parents should do everything they can to keep their children from experiencing stress.

Stress can have a negative impact on a child's behavior and even their perceptions of things. How does stress affect children?

Stress and children

1. Stress affects children's mental development.

Research shows that children who face stressful situations are more likely to experience problems in their mental development. When a child is stressed, challenges arise. In school, children cannot concentrate on their studies. Their concentration can also be affected, which can affect their overall performance in school.

2. Stress can dramatically change children's behavior.

Young people who experience stress at home and at school will tend to have dramatic changes in their behavior. One of the most obvious results is that children who are under great stress will stay away from other people and are distant. They tend to lack self-confidence and avoid socializing with others.

Some children suffering from stressful situations may experience low self-esteem. This affects the way they interact with other people and the way they see themselves.

3. Stress can affect their eating habits.

To ensure your child's growth and development, you must provide foods with complete nutrition. In addition to providing healthy meals, you should also ensure that your children do not experience stress at home. When a child is stressed, their eating habits can change. Some will tend to overeat, which can later lead to obesity, while other children will lose their appetite and not eat.

When this happens, their overall growth and development will be greatly affected. Without complete nutrition and all the stress they have to endure, children may experience health problems and other health risks associated with stress.

How can children avoid stress?

Unlike adults who have to live and cope with the world on their own, children are protected by their families and other loved ones.

No matter how innocent and young they are, they should not be faced with stressful situations that can negatively affect their attitude, behavior, and even their character in the long run.

As a parent, it is your obligation to ensure that your children grow up in a peaceful, safe and stress-free environment. Of course, stressful situations cannot be totally avoided. But as a parent, you must do everything you can to protect your children while they are still young.

After all, they don't know much about the complicated issues around them.

Chapter 8: Helping Young People De-stress

Young people at some point in their lives may experience stress. This is something that parents and children cannot avoid. For example, when a child sees his or her parents arguing or fighting, it can be really stressful. When children experience problems at school, they can also cause stress.

Parents cannot completely avoid and protect their children from stressful situations. But what you can do is find ways to help your children de-stress. When a child is under stress, it is important to have a strong support group.

What are the different ways to help your children de-stress?

How to help

1. Importance of communication

Many parents, with their busy schedules and other obligations, tend to forget the importance of communication. Although they attend to their children's needs, some spend little time asking how their children are doing in school or how they are doing. Without contact communication, children can feel alone. When something bad happens or when they experience any stressful situation, they will definitely have a hard time dealing with the problem. They don't want to share it with other people.

That's why it's crucial for parents to communicate constantly with their children. When children talk to their parents, they can share their thoughts and feelings. If they feel any stress, they don't have to carry the burden alone. Their parents can definitely comfort them.

2. Make time for your children

Family relationships are also very important, especially because young people have to deal with certain stages of growth and development when they may have to face difficult situations that are very stressful for them. Therefore, it is essential that children do not feel alone on this journey.

Parents must always show their children how much they love and care for them. No matter how busy you are, you should always look for ways to reach out and connect with your children. Even with your busy schedule, you should have time to bond with them and show them how important they are. When children feel loved at home, they can get through difficult situations easily.

3. Ensuring good health

For your children to be active and vibrant in school, you need to make sure that all their needs are met, especially with regard to their overall health. Prepare meals that boost their energy and sharpen their minds.

Children who eat nutritious meals and those who have the full daily requirement of vitamins and minerals are less likely to suffer from stress.

Getting plenty of sleep is also an important factor. When a child barely gets enough sleep, the tendency is for him to become easily irritated. Make sure your children get an early night and a full night's sleep.

4. Grace Under Pressure

Children tend to follow what they normally see. Their parents' behavior and attitude toward certain events or instances may influence how children cope with clothing.

Therefore, when parents are faced with stressful situations, they need to handle any problem with grace.

Chapter 9: New Technology for Children's Health

Technology has brought about significant changes not only for adults but also for children.

When you go to different stores, you will notice that there is a great variety of modern products that your children will surely love and enjoy.

Apart from the entertainment value that technology can give your child, there are also other aspects of your child's growth and development where technology can be a good contributor.

In relating new technology to health, how can you use available technology to improve your child's overall health? Is it really possible to use technology for children's health?

The answer is a big "Yes!

With advances in technology, there are now ways to develop the different aspects of your children's health.

These include the following:

New Technology

Mental Health

One of the aspects that can be further developed with the use of technology is mental health. Today, many children are more competitive and more intelligent. They can easily operate different types of devices and appliances. For parents, now is the time to make use of today's technology.

For example, parents who want to sharpen their children's memory and expand their imagination can allow their children to play different types of games online. Through a portable device, young people can enjoy various types of games in which they have the opportunity to use their brain and think about certain strategies. In addition, they can also interact and socialize with other children who are also playing the same game.

But, of course, parents should continue to guide their children whenever they spend time using these devices for educational purposes.

Physical Health

Another aspect of health that can be worked on with the use of technology is physical health. With so many products available to children, they can choose which specific items they want to have to improve their physical health.

There are now play devices where children have the opportunity to exercise and move their bodies. They can dance and play different sports without having to go outside, as there are play devices that allow them to perform these functions. Not only can they enjoy themselves but they can also exercise without being aware that they are exercising.

Oral Health

Kids love to eat candy. From candy to chocolates, it's not so easy to control their appetite when it comes to sweets.

Although parents can control the foods and food products their children eat, there are still cases where they cannot.

The result is that some children, if not all, suffer from significant dental health problems. Some experience tooth decay.

But thanks to technology, there are now several dental services along with different dental treatments and procedures to ensure that your children have a complete set of bright, white teeth.

Dentists now make use of today's technology to prevent any cavities and help children have good teeth.

Chapter 10: The benefits of teaching young people about good health

At a very early age, you can already lay the foundation for ensuring your children's good health. Even if they don't fully understand everything you want to do, at least you have the opportunity to guide them. The foods they eat can definitely impact their overall growth and development.

As a parent, you can raise your children in a way that gives them the correct and complete nutrition and provides a safe and healthy environment in which to grow. There are long-term benefits to teaching young people about good health.

The benefits

1. Develop the right habits.

Many adults who tend to have a sedentary lifestyle often have bad eating habits. Not only do they lack exercise, but some would prefer to eat foods that contain too much fat, salt, and sugar. Some would smoke or drink alcohol. All of this can be attributed in large part to the kind of habits they may have developed when they were young.

This is basically one of the reasons why it is important that while children are still young, they start forming good habits. For example, you should not allow your children to eat foods that are not nutritionally sound. When your children prefer to eat vegetables and fruits, they will carry on these good habits even when they are older.

2.   Ensure your child's growth and development.

Guiding your child to develop the right habits is only one aspect. When parents teach their children the importance of good health, they are also ensuring their children's development. The foods children eat can have a positive or negative impact on their growth. If parents allow children to eat what they want without making sure they have all the nutrients, then this can negatively affect children's growth.

3. The foundation and essential elements of good health are established.

In addition to encouraging your children to have good eating habits, you also lay the foundation for good health.

One obvious example is that when your child starts being physically active in sports at an early stage, he or she can maintain that attitude later on.

This is why it is strongly recommended that if children like a particular sport, parents should encourage their children to participate in their chosen sport.

4. Children can decrease stressful encounters.

When a child is in good health, they can avoid stress compared to other children. Remember that the foods your children eat, their meetings and daily activities can add stress.

But if your child eats nutritious foods and exercises regularly, he or she is expected to easily avoid stress.

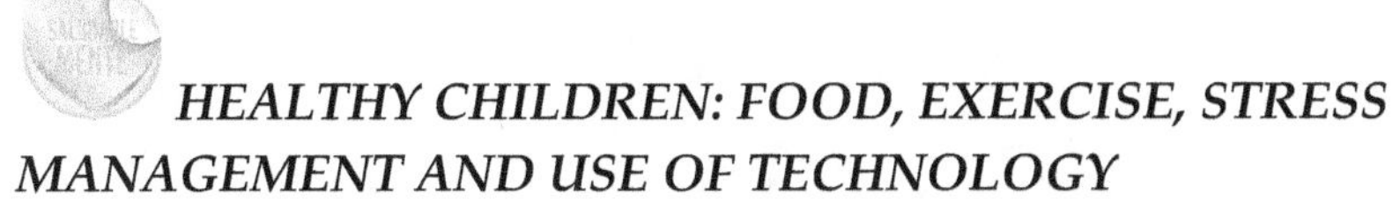

Ending

Helping your child develop the right habits and laying the groundwork for exploring health in general can have long-term benefits. As a parent, it is YOUR duty and obligation to provide the best kind of life you can give. At least, when your child grows up and starts to grow up, they will always remember the things they have been taught!

SUCCESS!